HERBAL REMEDIES FOR HERPES

Unlocking Nature's Healing Power For Targeting Relief, Holistic Wellness, Immune Support And Integrating Herbs Into Your Wellness Routine

DR. CARDEN KYRIE

DISCLAIMER

The only goal of this book is informational. Every effort has been taken by the author and publisher to ensure that the information provided is accurate. But the material in this book is given "as is," without any express or implied representation, warranty, or condition as to its accuracy, completeness, or suitability for any particular purpose.

Any loss, damage, or injury resulting from using the information in this book, or from any action or decision made as a result of such use, will not be covered by the author's or publisher's liability. It is recommended that readers seek the assistance of a certified specialist for guidance specific to their situation.

The opinions and viewpoints conveyed in this book belong to the author and may not necessarily represent the official stance or policies of any specified organizations or people. Any likeness to real-life occurrences, places, or people—living or deceased—is wholly coincidental.

No specific product, service, or therapy discussed in this book is endorsed by the author or publisher. Any reference to goods or services is made only for informative reasons and is not intended as a recommendation or endorsement.

Before making any judgments or acting on any information, readers are urged to independently confirm it all. Any unfavorable effects or repercussions arising from the usage of the material included in this book are disclaimed by the author and publisher.

By using this book, you consent to absolving the publisher and author of any and all claims, obligations, or losses resulting from your use of the material in it.

I appreciate your cooperation and understanding.

TABLE OF CONTENTS

INTRODUCTION TO HERPES
OVERVIEW AND HISTORY OF HERPES

Herpes simplex virus (HSV), which is mostly divided into two types: HSV-1 and HSV-2, is the virus that causes herpes. HSV-2 causes genital herpes, but HSV-1 is mainly linked to oral herpes, which appears as fever blisters or cold sores. Herpes viruses, both varieties, are extremely contagious and can spread by direct skin-to-body contact or bodily fluid contact with an infected individual. The virus causes repeated outbreaks of symptoms and stays in the body for life once it has been infected.

Beyond just the physical symptoms of the infection, herpes affects people emotionally and socially. The stigma associated with herpes can cause anxiety, loneliness, and feelings of humiliation. Furthermore, the repeated nature of breakouts presents continuous difficulties for individuals infected with the virus, affecting their quality of life.

THE VALUE OF NATURAL TREATMENTS

Considering the complex nature of herpes, the book lays a strong focus on the value of using natural therapies in addition to or instead of traditional medical treatments. Natural therapies are investigated for their ability to improve overall well-being, support the immune system, and relieve symptoms. These remedies include dietary adjustments, herbal supplements, and lifestyle alterations.

Natural medicine has a long history of use and is becoming more widely acknowledged in modern medicine for its all-encompassing and frequently softer methods. The goal of the book is to assist readers in investigating herbal therapies that could help control the symptoms of herpes, lessen the frequency of outbreaks, and enhance overall quality of life.

CHAPTER ONE

COMPREHENDING HERPES

DIFFERENT HERPES VIRUS TYPES

Herpesviruses are DNA viruses that belong to the Herpesviridae family and cause a range of viral illnesses known as herpes. Herpes viruses come in various varieties, each with unique traits and clinical presentations. The most well-known ones include Varicella-Zoster Virus (VZV), Herpes Simplex Virus Type 2 (HSV-2), and Herpes Simplex Virus Type 1 (HSV-1).

TYPE 1 HERPES SIMPLEX VIRUS (HSV-1)

HSV-1 is frequently linked to oral herpes, which can result in fever blisters or cold sores on the face and lips. It is mainly spread by oral-to-oral contact and is extremely contagious. Many people become infected with HSV-1 after being exposed to it as children, and infections are common.

The virus creates latent infections in nerve cells, which can result in repeated outbreaks at any point in an individual's lifetime. Even though oral herpes is usually seen as a moderate infection, people with weakened immune systems may experience more severe symptoms and discomfort from the infection.

TYPE 2 HERPES SIMPLEX VIRUS (HSV-2)

Conversely, genital herpes is a sexually transmitted infection primarily caused by HSV-2. The development of painful sores or ulcers in the vaginal and anal areas is the hallmark of genital herpes. Sexual interaction with an infected individual can spread HSV-2 and cause recurring outbreaks. Similar to HSV-1, the virus causes nerve cells to go into latency, which permits sporadic reactivation. Because of its effects on sexual health and the possibility of spreading to partners or newborns after childbirth, genital herpes can be a serious worry.

VIRUS VARICELLA-ZOSTER (VZV)

The varicella-zoster virus, or VZV, causes both shingles and chickenpox, two different clinical entities. The symptoms of chickenpox, which usually affects children, include a widespread rash and itchy skin sores. The virus stays dormant in nerve cells after a person recovers from chickenpox and may resurface as shingles later in life. Shingles commonly affects one side of the body and manifests as a painful rash with blisters filled with fluid. Shingles are more common in older people and those with compromised immune systems.

In contrast to HSV-1 and HSV-2, VZV is predominantly transmitted by respiratory droplets rather than being linked to sexually transmitted illnesses.

It is essential to comprehend the various herpes virus kinds for efficient administration, diagnosis, and prevention. Herpes infections are incurable, however, antiviral drugs might help manage symptoms and lessen the frequency of outbreaks.

The impact of these infections on people and communities can be reduced with the use of safe behaviors, regular medical screenings, and public awareness campaigns.

CHAPTER TWO
RISK AND TRANSMISSION FACTORS
SEXUAL TRANSMISSION

Not just sexually transmitted infections (STIs), but also other infectious diseases, are mostly conveyed through sexual contact. During sexual practices, such as vaginal, anal, or oral intercourse, infections can spread from one person to another through the exchange of bodily fluids. STDs that are frequently contracted include chlamydia, syphilis, gonorrhea, and HIV. The existence of open sores, the use of preventative measures like condoms, and an individual's general sexual health habits all have an impact on the risk of transmission. Reducing the risk of sexual transmission requires regular screenings and education on safe sex practices.

NON-SEXUAL TRANSMISSION

Contrary to sexual transmission, non-sexual methods can also be used to spread infectious diseases. These pathways include eating contaminated food or water, breathing in infected droplets, coming into direct touch with contaminated surfaces or objects, and vector-borne transmission via insects like ticks or mosquitoes. A multitude of infections, from the common cold to more serious ailments like influenza and COVID-19, are transmitted through non-sexual means. To stop the spread of diseases within communities and prevent non-sexual transmission of disease, it is essential to understand and put into practice appropriate hygiene habits, vaccinations, and infection control measures.

DIAGNOSIS AND SYMPTOMS

Depending on the type of infectious agent, there are considerable variations in how symptoms present. Fever, exhaustion, coughing, respiratory discomfort, gastrointestinal problems, and skin manifestations are some of the common symptoms. Differentiating between infections that share similar first symptoms can be difficult. A prompt and precise diagnosis is essential to the successful management and containment of the illness. To determine the cause, medical practitioners use a variety of techniques, such as imaging examinations, laboratory testing, and clinical evaluations. In rare circumstances, the presence of particular antigens or antibodies in blood samples may help with diagnosis confirmation.

COMMON SYMPTOMS

Due to the large variety of microorganisms that can cause illness, the symptoms of infectious diseases can vary greatly. Anemia and lethargy are frequently present with fever, which is a defining feature of numerous illnesses. Symptoms of respiratory infections might include coughing, dyspnea, and soreness in the chest. Abdominal pain, vomiting, and diarrhea can all be symptoms of gastrointestinal illnesses. Rashes, sores, or lesions are some of the symptoms of skin infections. It's critical to identify these typical symptoms to provide early detection and timely medical attention. It is important to remember, though, that the absence of symptoms does not always mean that an infection is not there. This is because many infections might have an incubation period before symptoms manifest or be asymptomatic.

DIAGNOSTIC TECHNIQUES

A variety of diagnostic techniques are used to determine the origin of infectious diseases. Clinical evaluations entail analyzing a patient's physical examination, medical history, and symptoms. Crucial diagnostics include blood tests, cultures, and molecular methods such as polymerase chain reaction (PCR) in the laboratory. Investigations using imaging tests, such as CT or X-rays, can shed light on internal organ infections. Serological tests can confirm specific infections by identifying antigens or antibodies in blood samples. The type of disease and the probable infection determine which diagnostic approach is best. Initiating appropriate treatment and putting public health measures in place to stop additional transmission requires a timely and accurate diagnosis.

CHAPTER THREE

TRADITIONAL HERPES TREATMENTS
ANTIVIRAL DRUGS

The mainstay of conventional herpes treatment is the use of antiviral drugs; Acyclovir, Valacyclovir, and Famciclovir are the three most often recommended medications. Both type 1 (HSV-1) and type 2 (HSV-2) herpes simplex virus infections are commonly treated with these drugs.

ACYCLOVIR

One of the first antiviral medications for herpes, acyclovir, has proved essential in treating this viral infection. It functions by preventing the viral enzyme DNA polymerase from acting, which restricts the herpes virus's ability to replicate. Acyclovir is available in a range of formulations to suit varying phases and severity of herpes outbreaks, such as oral pills, intravenous injections, and topical creams.

VALACYCLOVIR

Another common herpes treatment prescribed is valacyclovir, an antiviral prodrug of acyclovir. After consumption, the body transforms Valacyclovir into Acyclovir. Compared to Acyclovir, this prodrug formulation has the benefit of greater bioavailability, which enables less frequent dosing. Because of this, valacyclovir is a practical and efficient choice for suppressive treatment against herpes outbreaks as well as episodic therapy.

FAMCICLOVIR

Another antiviral drug in the same class as valacyclovir and acyclovir is famciclovir. After consumption, it is changed into penciclovir, which is its active form. Like Acyclovir, penciclovir inhibits the replication of viral DNA. Those seeking oral antiviral medication may find famciclovir to be an appealing alternative due to its simple dosing regimen and special effectiveness in treating recurrent genital herpes outbreaks.

The best results from these antiviral drugs come from starting them early in a herpes epidemic. They are frequently given during active outbreaks as part of episodic treatment, which lessens the intensity and duration of symptoms. Antiviral therapy can also be utilized as a suppressive treatment for people who experience severe or frequent recurrences. In these situations, taking the drug daily helps to either avoid or lessen the frequency of breakouts.

Antiviral drugs can effectively control symptoms and lessen the frequency of outbreaks, but they cannot treat herpes. This is crucial to remember. Although these medications lessen the symptoms, control the virus, and lower the chance of transmission, the virus still exists in the body latently and may occasionally reactivate.

Antiviral drugs are usually well tolerated, although some people may experience negative effects. Symptoms such as headaches, nausea, and stomach pain are frequently experienced. Before beginning antiviral therapy, patients with specific medical conditions or those on other medications should speak with their healthcare provider to be sure the treatment is safe and effective for them.

Antiviral drugs like Acyclovir, Valacyclovir, and Famciclovir are essential to the traditional management of herpes. These medications help people with herpes infections manage their symptoms effectively, lessen the frequency of outbreaks, and improve their general quality of life.

CHAPTER FOUR

OTC (OVER-THE-COUNTER) DRUGS

PAIN-RELIEVING AGENTS

An important class of over-the-counter (OTC) drugs is pain relievers, which provide non-prescription pain relief for a range of pain types and intensities. Nonsteroidal anti-inflammatory drugs (NSAIDs), including ibuprofen and naproxen, which decrease pain and inflammation by blocking specific enzymes, are commonly included in these prescriptions. Another popular over-the-counter pain treatment that is frequently suggested for people who are allergic to or have stomach problems and cannot take NSAIDs is acetaminophen.

To provide momentary respite, pain medications function by preventing the body from producing molecules that indicate pain. Nonetheless, people must follow prescribed dosage recommendations to prevent adverse consequences, such as liver damage from acetaminophen overuse.

TOPICAL LOTIONS

Another class of over-the-counter (OTC) drugs for pain relief are topical creams. These creams, which are created with substances like menthol, camphor, or NSAIDs, are placed directly onto the skin. They are appropriate for ailments like arthritis, muscle aches, or joint pain because of their localized application, which enables tailored alleviation. Because they are convenient and don't have the systemic adverse effects that come with oral drugs, topical creams are preferred. Although they might provide some relief for mild to moderate pain, their efficacy varies, and people with sensitive skin should be aware of the possibility of adverse skin responses.

Topical creams and over-the-counter pain medications have advantages in terms of accessibility and convenience, but they are not without drawbacks. First and foremost, instead of treating the fundamental source of the pain, they are frequently made to manage its symptoms. This implies that although they might offer some respite, they might not be a permanent fix for long-term ailments. To prevent possible interactions or negative effects, people with specific medical problems or those taking other medications should speak with a healthcare provider before using over-the-counter pain remedies.

CONSEQUENCES AND RESTRICTIONS OF TRADITIONAL THERAPIES

Additionally, each person may react differently to over-the-counter drugs, and some may not get the relief they need. Furthermore, overuse or continuous use of over-the-counter painkillers, particularly NSAIDs, can have negative consequences like bleeding in the stomach, kidney troubles, or heart difficulties. Users must be informed about possible adverse effects and seek medical advice if their pain worsens or if they have any concerns.

Topical creams and over-the-counter painkillers are essential for treating different kinds of pain. Although they are easily accessible and convenient, users should be aware of the limitations, possible adverse effects, and dose recommendations of these traditional remedies. For those with underlying medical issues or chronic pain, seeking professional advice is essential to ensuring safe and efficient pain treatment.

CHAPTER FIVE

NATURAL METHODS FOR TREATING HERPES

NUTRITIONAL ADJUSTMENTS

Dietary adjustments are important for the natural management of herpes since they strengthen the immune system and reduce risk factors for outbreaks. Stressing the need for a healthy, well-balanced diet is essential for maintaining general health and building resistance to the herpes simplex virus (HSV). Managing symptoms and lowering the frequency of breakouts can be achieved by including some meals and avoiding others.

FOODS TO INCLUDE

People with herpes must eat a diet high in nutrients that strengthen the immune system. Citrus fruits, strawberries, and bell peppers are good sources of vitamin C, which is well known for boosting immunity. In a similar vein, foods rich in antioxidants, such as almonds, berries, and leafy green vegetables, can assist the body's defense mechanisms and fight oxidative stress.

The amino acid lysine has been researched for its ability to prevent the herpes virus from replicating. Lysine-rich foods include fish, poultry, eggs, and dairy products. Furthermore, because zinc is involved in immune function, foods high in zinc, such as beans, lentils, and seeds, may be advantageous.

Consuming omega-3 fatty acids, which are present in flaxseeds and fatty fish like salmon, may have anti-inflammatory properties and help control the symptoms of herpes. Foods high in probiotics, such as yogurt and fermented foods, help improve gut health, which is associated with better immune function.

FOODS TO AVOID

It's best to limit your intake of certain foods since they may aggravate your herpes symptoms or cause outbreaks. Whole grains, nuts, seeds, chocolate, and other high-protein foods include large amounts of arginine, an amino acid that facilitates the herpes virus. Even though these foods are usually nutritious, those who have herpes might benefit from consuming them in moderation.

To assist in keeping the ratio in the desired range, foods high in lysine and foods high in arginine should be balanced in the diet. Reducing the intake of processed meals, sugary snacks, and alcohol is also advised because these items might weaken immune systems and increase inflammation, which may lead to herpes outbreaks.

Keeping up a nutritious and well-balanced diet is just one facet of managing herpes naturally. People must seek individualized advice from healthcare specialists and include dietary modifications in a holistic approach to controlling the condition.

HERBAL TREATMENTS

Herbal treatments are commonly used in natural approaches to managing herpes because they are thought to have antiviral and immune-boosting qualities. Among these cures, aloe vera, lemon balm, and echinacea have become well-known due to their supposed ability to assist the body's defense mechanisms and reduce symptoms.

ECHINACEA

The plant echinacea, which is derived from the coneflower, is well known for activating the immune system. It is thought to strengthen the body's defenses against infections, such as the herpes virus. Alkamides and polysaccharides, which are abundant in echinacea, may be involved in the plant's antiviral properties. Echinacea pills or extracts, according to some supporters, may help regulate the immune system and maybe lessen the frequency or intensity of herpes outbreaks.

LEMON BALM

There is also a history of traditional use of lemon balm, or Melissa officinalis, in the management of herpes symptoms. Citronellal and geranial, two of the essential oils present in lemon balm, are thought to have antiviral qualities. Based on research, topical application of a lemon balm cream or ointment may speed up the healing process of herpes lesions and ease related pain. Furthermore, lemon balm's relaxing properties might benefit stress, which is known to be a herpes outbreak cause.

ALOE VERA

Succulent aloe vera is a plant with several medicinal uses that are frequently linked to good skin. Aloe Vera is well known for its ability to relieve burns and wounds, but some supporters claim it can also help control the symptoms of herpes. Bioactive substances found in the gel made from Aloe Vera leaves include glycoproteins and polysaccharides, which are thought to have immune-modulating and antiviral qualities. Herpes lesions may heal more quickly and experience less inflammation and itching if Aloe Vera gel is applied topically.

It is imperative to acknowledge that although herbal medicines such as Aloe Vera, Lemon Balm, and Echinacea may have potential advantages, their effectiveness may differ across individuals. Furthermore, there isn't much scientific data to support the usage of these herbs specifically for managing herpes; further studies are required to definitively prove their efficacy. To verify safety and talk about any drug interactions, people are urged to speak with healthcare providers before implementing herbal therapies into a herpes management strategy.

Herbal treatments including aloe vera, lemon balm, and echinacea are a few of the natural strategies investigated for herpes management. Although these herbs have been utilized historically for their possible immune-modulating and antiviral properties, it is important to use caution when using them. Although there is still much to learn about the efficacy of these herbal treatments for managing herpes, people should speak with medical specialists for specific advice and to make sure incorporating these remedies into their routine is in line with their general health and well-being.

TEA TREE LIQUID

Essential oils are concentrated plant extracts with medicinal qualities that are frequently used in natural herpes control techniques. Tea tree oil is unique among essential oils that have received attention for managing herpes because of its antiviral and antibacterial qualities. It has been discovered that substances like terpinene-4-ol, which are extracted from the leaves of the Melaleuca alternifolia tree, have antiviral properties. Although there isn't much study on tea tree oil specifically for herpes, anyone looking into natural therapies may find it interesting due to its broad antiviral qualities.

OIL OF LAVENDER

Another essential oil that's frequently used in the natural treatment of herpes is lavender oil. Linalool and linalyl acetate are two substances found in lavender that contribute to its antiviral and anti-inflammatory qualities, as well as its pleasing aroma and relaxing qualities. While further research is required to determine the effectiveness of lavender oil especially for herpes, some people use it in their holistic practices because they think it may help with symptoms and improve general health.

OIL OF PEPPERMINT

The leaves of the Mentha piperita plant are used to make peppermint oil, which is known to have some advantages in naturally treating herpes symptoms. It has menthol, which has anti-inflammatory and antiviral qualities. Although there isn't any concrete research supporting peppermint oil's effectiveness in treating herpes, people looking for complementary therapies frequently choose it for its calming and cooling properties. According to some supporters, peppermint oil may help reduce the discomfort and itching brought on by herpes outbreaks.

When it comes to essential oils, it's important to stress that although these natural remedies could have certain advantages, they shouldn't be used as stand-alone treatments for herpes. People should use caution when using essential oils as therapies for herpes because there is now little scientific data to support their efficacy. Before using essential oils in a herpes management program, it is best to speak with medical authorities, particularly if the patient is using prescription drugs or has a history of medical issues.

Essential oils are frequently applied topically to afflicted regions after being diluted with carrier oils for herpes treatment. However, as essential oils are very concentrated chemicals, one must be aware of the possibility of skin irritation or allergic responses.

It's a good idea to conduct a patch test on a tiny patch of skin before using something widely.

Essential oils such as peppermint, lavender, and tea tree have drawn interest due to their possible application in the natural treatment of herpes. Even though some people have had success with these treatments, it is important to approach their use cautiously in light of the scant scientific data. Comprehensive management of herpes requires consulting with healthcare professionals and using a holistic strategy that incorporates lifestyle variables, antiviral drugs (if required), and medical advice.

CHAPTER SIX

BEHAVIORAL AND LIFESTYLE STRATEGIES

HANDLING STRESS:

Today's environment is demanding and fast-paced, making stress an inevitable component of day-to-day existence. Maintaining general well-being and avoiding the detrimental effects of long-term stress on physical and mental health depend on effective stress management. A crucial component of stress management is learning coping skills to get through difficult circumstances. This can involve prioritizing work, identifying and changing cognitive habits, and creating attainable goals. Stress reduction can also be greatly aided by creating a supportive social network and getting expert assistance when necessary.

PRACTICE MEDITATION

A centuries-old discipline, meditation has become more popular in modern society as a means of fostering emotional equilibrium, cerebral clarity, and general well-being. Through guided or silent sessions, one can cultivate a heightened state of awareness and focus as part of this mindfulness method. Frequent meditation has been linked to a host of advantages, such as lowered stress levels, increased emotional well-being, and better concentration. People can choose from a variety of meditation styles, including transcendental meditation and mindfulness meditation, to fit their interests and lifestyles.

BREATHING TECHNIQUES

Exercises for deep breathing sometimes referred to as diaphragmatic or abdominal breathing, are easy yet powerful ways to ease tension and encourage relaxation. In these exercises, the diaphragm is fully expanded through a deliberate and gradual inhale through the nose, which is followed by a controlled exhale through the mouth. By inducing a state of relaxation in the body, deep breathing lowers stress hormones and activates the parasympathetic nervous system. Deep breathing can be used as a quick fix for stressful situations or incorporated into daily routines to produce immediate calming effects. People of all ages can participate in this activity, which can be easily incorporated into a variety of lifestyles.

All things considered, including stress-reduction methods into one's daily routine, such as deep breathing exercises and meditation, can promote equilibrium and fortitude in the face of adversity. These activities are essential for fostering long-term mental and physical well-being in addition to helping with short-term stress alleviation. People who practice mindfulness in handling stress are more equipped to deal with the complexity of contemporary life and bounce back from setbacks.

SUITABLE SLEEP POSITION

The term "sleep hygiene" describes a collection of behaviors and routines that support restful sleep. It entails setting up a space and making lifestyle choices that support sound sleep. This entails establishing a relaxing sleep environment, practicing relaxation techniques before bedtime, and adhering to a regular sleep schedule. Enhancing the length and quality of sleep is the aim of sleep hygiene, which promotes general health.

THE VALUE OF GETTING ENOUGH SLEEP

Getting enough sleep is essential for preserving the best possible physical and mental health. Sleep is essential for several processes, including the immune system, memory consolidation, and emotional control. A higher risk of chronic illnesses like obesity, diabetes, and cardiovascular diseases has been associated with inadequate sleep. Furthermore, mood stability, productivity, and cognitive function all depend on getting enough sleep. Ensuring that you get the necessary amount of sleep regularly can make a big difference in your overall quality of life.

SUGGESTIONS FOR INCREASING SLEEP QUALITY

A few useful suggestions will help you get a better night's sleep. Essential sleep practices include sticking to a regular sleep schedule, making your bedroom cozy and dark, and avoiding stimulants like caffeine right before bed. Before going to bed, using relaxation methods like deep breathing exercises or meditation can also help reduce stress. Reducing the amount of time spent on screens before bed and establishing a relaxing ritual before bed can help the body know when it's time to relax. Creating and upholding these routines might help you get a better, more peaceful sleep that will revitalize you.

PHYSICAL ACTIVITY AND EXERCISE

Physical activity and regular exercise are essential parts of a healthy lifestyle. Exercise has a significant impact on mental health in addition to improving physical fitness. It has been connected to better mood, increased cognitive performance, and a lower chance of developing chronic illnesses. Regular physical activity is linked to higher-quality sleep, so it's a useful tactic for people trying to enhance their sleep habits in general.

ADVANTAGES OF FREQUENT EXERCISE

Frequent exercise has advantages that go beyond improved physical health. Exercise has been demonstrated to lower stress, anxiety, and sadness by encouraging the body's natural mood enhancers, endorphins, to be released. It also contributes to better cardiovascular health and managing weight. Moreover, regular exercise improves the quality of sleep by facilitating quicker sleep onset and deeper, more restorative slumber.

EXERCISES THAT ARE GOOD FOR PEOPLE WITH HERPES

Regular exercise is often safe and useful for people who have herpes. But it's crucial to pick low-impact pursuits and stay away from situations that could make symptoms worse. Exercises like yoga, swimming, and walking are typically well-tolerated. It is best to speak with medical experts to find an exercise program that fits specific medical needs and takes care of any herpes-related issues. Exercise regimens should be customized to each person's demands and limits to maximize the health benefits of physical activity for people with herpes while lowering any dangers.

CHAPTER SEVEN

SUPPORT FOR THE IMMUNE SYSTEM

VITAMIN C IS A NUTRITIONAL SUPPLEMENT

Nutritional supplements are essential for boosting immunity and promoting general well-being as well as resistance to illness. Of these supplements, vitamin C is particularly important. Due to its well-known antioxidant qualities, vitamin C aids in the fight against inflammation and oxidative stress, two conditions that are critical to immune function. Additionally, Vitamin C encourages the development of white blood cells, key components of the immune system responsible for fighting off infections.

ZINC

Zinc is another key vitamin for immune system support. It plays a vital role in several immunological processes, including the stimulation of T cells and the generation of antibodies. Zinc insufficiency has been related to poor immunological responses, making it vital to ensure an appropriate intake of this mineral for healthy immune function.

LYSINE

Lysine, an important amino acid, is recognized for its potential to strengthen the immune system. It is involved in the development of antibodies and has been examined for its capacity to block the replication of some viruses. Including lysine-rich foods or supplements in the diet may contribute to a robust immune response.

PROBIOTICS AND INTESTINAL HEALTH

Probiotics, helpful microorganisms that create a healthy gut microbiome, are increasingly recognized for their immune-modulating effects. The gut is a crucial participant in immune system function, and maintaining its health is paramount. Probiotics improve the balance of intestinal flora, boosting the body's ability to respond to diseases effectively.

IMPORTANCE OF A HEALTHY GUT

The importance of a healthy gut cannot be emphasized in the context of immune system support. The gut is home to a substantial amount of the body's immune cells and functions as a barrier against hazardous invaders. A robust immune system is supported by a diversified and well-balanced microbiome, which helps to limit overreaction to benign stimuli and encourages a suitable reaction to real threats.

FOODS HIGH IN PROBIOTICS

Foods high in probiotics are a great natural method to improve gut health. Probiotic-rich foods including kefir, yogurt, sauerkraut, kimchi, and other fermented foods enter the digestive tract. These microorganisms support immunological function by preserving the gut microbiota's equilibrium. Consuming a range of foods high in probiotics can help maintain a healthy gut environment.

Nutritional supplements play a critical part in the comprehensive approach to immune system support. Probiotics and preserving gut health lay the groundwork for general immunological resilience, while zinc, lysine, and vitamin C directly affect immune function. A strong and efficient immune response can be facilitated by including a variety of nutrient-rich foods and supplements in one's diet, which will enhance general health and well-being.

CHAPTER EIGHT

COMBINING MEDICAL CARE WITH NATURAL SOLUTIONS

TALKING WITH MEDICAL PROFESSIONALS

A careful and cooperative approach is required when combining natural therapies with medical care, with communication with healthcare professionals acting as a vital first step. People should have open lines of communication with their healthcare providers before starting any integrative plan to make sure they fully understand their medical history, present symptoms, and any ongoing therapies.

This cooperative consultation enables a comprehensive evaluation, assisting medical professionals in assisting patients in making decisions on the integration of natural therapies.

INTEGRATING ANTIVIRAL DRUGS WITH NATURAL REMEDIES

Combining natural remedies with antiviral drugs is one area of particular interest when thinking about how to integrate natural remedies with medical therapies. Antiviral drugs are frequently administered to treat viral infections; however, to improve their immune system or reduce symptoms, patients may also look for complementary or alternative therapies. But be careful when integrating natural therapies with antiviral medications—some of them may interact negatively. To ensure that the combined approach is safe and effective while decreasing the potential of unwanted responses, consulting with healthcare specialists becomes crucial.

TRACKING AND MODIFYING TREATMENT PROGRAMS

A crucial component of the integration process is the monitoring and modification of treatment programs, which provide a flexible and individualized approach to healthcare. Frequent follow-ups with medical professionals enable evaluation of the integrated treatment strategy's overall efficacy. Monitoring is keeping an eye on how the patient responds to both conventional and complementary therapies, taking into account any alterations in symptoms, adverse effects, or other pertinent variables. Based on these evaluations, modifications to the treatment plan might be required to keep the integrative approach customized to the patient's changing health needs.

The possibility for interactions between various therapeutic modalities and the heterogeneity of individual reactions present one of the problems in integrating natural medicines with conventional treatment. Healthcare professionals are essential in enabling this integration because they use their knowledge to weigh the advantages and disadvantages. The cooperative character of the patient-provider interaction encourages shared decision-making, enabling people to take an active role in their healthcare journey and gain from the combined expertise of complementary and conventional methods.

Combining natural therapies with medical care is a complex process that calls for constant observation, open communication, and well-informed decision-making. A strong basis for this integration is created by consultation with medical professionals, who guarantee that the natural cures selected enhance rather than undermine traditional medical treatments. The prudent blending of herbal medicines with antiviral drugs necessitates close consideration of possible interactions, underscoring the value of expert advice. The efficacy of integrated healthcare solutions is eventually improved by a responsive and individualized approach made possible by regular monitoring and the flexibility to modify treatment regimens.

CHAPTER NINE

STOPPING HERPES EPIDEMICS

GUIDELINES FOR SAFE SEXUAL PRACTICES

Safe sexual behavior is essential for reducing the risk of transmission and averting herpes outbreaks. Using barrier techniques, like condoms, correctly and consistently is crucial during sexual activity, particularly if one partner has a history of herpes. By acting as a physical barrier, condoms can greatly lower the risk of the virus spreading. Condoms are very efficient, but it's crucial to remember that they don't offer complete protection because they might not cover every region that could be contaminated.

It's also critical that sexual partners communicate regularly. Making educated judgments about sexual activity can be aided by having candid conversations about each other's sexual health, including any history of herpes or other STIs. To foster an atmosphere where both parties feel comfortable sharing their status and talking about preventive actions, partners should be sympathetic and supportive.

CONTROLLING STRESS TO STOP OUTBREAKS

Since stress is known to be a trigger for herpes outbreaks, managing stress is essential to avoid recurrences. Herpes patients should learn several stress-reduction strategies to keep their emotional health and reduce the chance of outbreaks. Deep breathing techniques, yoga, and mindfulness meditation are a few practices that can help lower stress levels all around.

Another crucial component of stress management is regular exercise. Engaging in physical activity improves immune system performance, and general health, and reduces stress. Long-term benefits of establishing a regular exercise regimen include reducing the risk of herpes outbreaks and enhancing resilience to stressors.

Developing a positive work-life balance and looking for social support are other essential stress-reduction techniques. Having a solid network of friends, family, or a counselor by your side can help you cope emotionally when things get hard. Adopting a lifestyle that places a high priority on mental health benefits general health and well-being in addition to preventing herpes breakouts.

EXTENDED LIFESTYLE MODIFICATIONS

Long-term herpes outbreak prevention requires adopting a healthy lifestyle. This involves eating a well-balanced diet full of nutrients that strengthen the immune system. Sufficient consumption of vitamins and minerals, particularly zinc, lysine, and vitamin C, might boost immunity and perhaps lessen outbreak frequency.

It is equally vital to get enough sleep, as sleep deprivation can impair immunity and make an individual more vulnerable to diseases. In addition to improving general health, maintaining a regular sleep schedule and emphasizing proper sleep hygiene can help stop herpes outbreaks.

Other lifestyle modifications that can help with herpes control include cutting back on alcohol intake and staying away from tobacco products. Tobacco and alcohol both weaken the immune system, increasing a person's vulnerability to epidemics. Consequently, cutting back on or giving up these substances can improve one's general health and well-being.

A comprehensive strategy that incorporates long-term lifestyle modifications, healthy stress management techniques, and safe sexual behaviors is necessary to avoid herpes breakouts. Individuals who have herpes can reduce the frequency and intensity of outbreaks while improving general health and well-being by adopting these measures into their daily lives.